CANDIDIASIS SOLUTION

A Comprehensive Guide To Understanding And Managing Yeast Overgrowth.

Unraveling the Mystery of Yeast-Related Health Issues

BY

DR. ELVIRA S. GRAVES

TABLE OF CONTENTS

Disclaimer

Introduction

I am thrilled to introduce you to "Candidiasis Solution: A Comprehensive Guide to Understanding and Managing Yeast Overgrowth," as a physician dedicated to deciphering health and wellness mysteries. In these pages, we set out on an excursion — one that rises above simple clinical information and digs into the unpredictable dance between our bodies and the pioneering microorganism known as Candida.

Historical Perspective on the
Candida Mystery Candida has been a formidable foe and a silent companion for centuries. Its presence inside us is all around as old as humankind itself. However, we have only recently begun to fully comprehend its impact on our health. Candidiasis — the excess of Candida species — has quietly tormented incalculable people, causing a horde of side effects that frequently resist simple findings.

The Battle with Candidiasis

Imagine sitting across from me and hearing a patient talk about fatigue, brain fog, digestive issues, frequent infections, and inexplicable mood swings. As a doctor, I've seen the anger on their faces as they struggled to find answers, made innumerable visits to specialists, and received a bewildering array of contradictory advice. Candidiasis has long been a formidable foe, often going unnoticed and wreaking havoc on one's physical and emotional health.

What You Can Expect to Get From

This Guide We bridge the gap between scientific comprehension and practical empowerment in "Candidiasis Solution." You, the reader, will gain the following:

1. Information: We demystify Candida — its life cycle, conduct, and effect on different body frameworks. You will be able to recognize the subtle signs and comprehend the intricate web of symptoms with this knowledge.

2. Demonstrative Clearness: We dig into symptomatic methodologies, furnishing you with the apparatuses to separate between intense and ongoing candidiasis. You will confidently navigate the diagnostic maze, including candida-specific assessments and laboratory tests.

3. Holistic Strategies: In addition to antifungal medications, we investigate stress management, dietary changes, and lifestyle

changes. You'll find how reestablishing stomach wellbeing and adjusting your microbiome can be strong partners in the battle against Candida.

4. Natural Remedies: Our guide offers suggestions for herbal supplements, probiotics, and topical treatments that are supported by evidence. These regular arrangements enable you to assume responsibility for your well-being.

5. Long haul Versatility: Anticipation is critical. We guide you in keeping a candida-safe way of life, checking side effects, and forestalling backslides. The present Answers for The upcoming Wellbeing Keep in mind that you are not alone as we move through these pages. Numerous lives have been shaped by candidiasis, as have the triumphs of those who recovered their vitality. Our main goal is clear: to engage you with information, sympathy, and significant stages. Use this as a beacon to help you find your way to resilience, harmony, and vibrant health. Welcome to "Candidiasis Arrangement." May it help you see the way to wellness and motivate you to regain your vitality.

[Dr. Elvira S. Graves]

Chapter 1: Understanding Candidiasis

Candidiasis, also known as a yeast infection, is a common fungal disease brought on by an excessive amount of Candida species. Our bodies naturally contain these microscopic fungi, particularly in the gastrointestinal tract, skin, and mucous membranes. However, candidiasis can occur if the delicate balance that exists between Candida and other microorganisms is disturbed. Candidiasis contamination frequently shows up on your skin, vagina, or mouth, where Candida normally resides in modest quantities. Solid microorganisms in your body forestall yeast abundance. Envision you have a two-outfitted scale with sound microorganisms on one side and yeast on the other. Until a disruption occurs as a result of stress, poor diet, a compromised immune system, or an uncontrolled medical condition, the scale remains level. A Candidiasis infection occurs when your scale is disrupted by something else. Because yeast lives naturally in our bodies and it is simple to upset the balance between healthy bacteria and yeast, candidiasis can affect anyone. Candidiasis can strike both healthy and immunocompromised individuals. Candidiasis most frequently influences: People who have diabetes, women who are pregnant, children, people who wear dentures, people who are in a hospital, and people who use a catheter Candidiasis is a typical condition. The most regular kind of candidiasis is a vaginal yeast disease, which influences around 75% of individuals with a vagina something like once in the course of their life. Albeit uncommon, serious instances of obtrusive candidiasis influence almost 25,000 people in the U.S. every year. Until you find treatment, candidiasis causes discomfort, itchiness, and irritation but does not pose a significant threat to your overall health. Like whatever other disease that you could get from a physical issue, it's ideal to treat the contamination at the primary sign to ease your side effects. Serious infections could spread to other parts of your body, including your blood, heart, and brain if candidiasis is not treated. candidiasis subtypes Because yeast lives naturally in your body, there are different kinds of candidiasis based on where the infection is located.

The following are candidiasis types:
A common infection that causes burning, itching, redness, and vaginal discharge is known as vaginal candidiasis (vaginitis); The vagina ordinarily contains a good arrangement of microorganisms and yeast. The chemical estrogen helps

microbes called lactobacilli to develop. These microorganisms kill hurtful life forms in the vagina and keep you sound. However, when something ends up tipping that equilibrium, a parasite called candida can outgrow control and cause a yeast disease, otherwise called vaginal candidiasis. No one likes to talk about them because they are itchy and uncomfortable.

In any case, vaginal yeast contaminations are extremely normal. 75% of women, according to estimates, will experience at least one yeast infection in their lifetime. However, yeast diseases can happen to anybody whenever certain things make them more probable. Most contaminations can be cleared up rapidly and without any problem. Compared to bacterial vaginosis, yeast infection Vaginal infections known as vaginitis include yeast infections and bacterial vaginosis (BV). While the circumstances might have comparative side effects, they occur for various reasons and need various medicines. You can involve an over-the-counter treatment for yeast contamination however will presumably require physician-recommended medication for BV.

Yeast contamination Causes
 There are many reasons you could get yeast contamination, including;

Hormones: Your vagina's hormonal balance can be affected by changes during pregnancy, breastfeeding, menopause, or taking birth control pills.

Diabetes: An increase in sugar in the vaginal mucous membranes can provide an environment for yeast growth if diabetes is not well controlled.

Anti-microbial: These medications can kill off large numbers of the great microorganisms that live in your vagina.

The use of vaginal sprays and douches can alter the balance in your vagina.

A weakened immune system: The yeast may also grow out of control if you are HIV-positive or have another immune system disorder.

Sex: However yeast contamination isn't viewed as a physically communicated disease, it tends to be passed from one individual to another through sexual contact.

The candida fungus, like other organisms, responds to stress, according to research. Our insight into this reaction for the most part comes from lab studies where researchers develop it in glucose. Yet, in the human body, growth faces various circumstances and is presented with many anxieties without a moment's delay, which affects its capacity to cause sickness.

Symptoms of a Yeast Infection

Irritation and distress are the primary side effects of a yeast disease, however, there are others: Copying, redness, and enlarging of the vagina and the vulva (the external piece of the female privates), Agony or copying when you pee, Agony during sex, A thick, white, scentless release, like curds, Watery release, Vaginal rash and Little cuts or minuscule breaks in the skin of your vulva.

Cutaneous candidiasis: A contamination on your skin that makes a raised, red fix with little, bothersome knocks that structure in folds of your skin, as in your underarms, under your bosoms, and close to your posterior (diaper rash) or crotch. Fungi frequently inhabit the hair, nails, and outer skin layers, which are the source of some fungal infections. They incorporate yeast-like parasites like candida. These yeast can sometimes get under the skin's surface and cause an infection. Candida fungi infect the skin in cutaneous candidiasis. This sort of disease is genuinely normal. It can affect almost any skin on the body, but the armpits and groin are the most common warm, moist, and creased areas. The organism that most frequently causes cutaneous candidiasis is Candida albicans. Candida is the most widely recognized reason for diaper rash in babies. The warm and moist conditions inside the diaper are used by the fungi. Additionally, diabetes and obesity are particularly common risk factors for Candida infection. Chemotherapy, steroids, and antibiotics all raise the risk of cutaneous candidiasis. Additionally, infections of the mouth's corners, edges, and nails can be brought on by Candida.

What Causes Skin Candidiasis?

When the skin becomes infected with Candida, it develops candidiasis. Candida fungi naturally reside on the skin in small quantities. However, infection can occur when this kind of fungus begins to multiply uncontrollably. This might happen due to: warm climate, tight dress, unfortunate cleanliness, rare underpants, changes, weight, the utilization of anti-infection agents that kill innocuous microbes that monitor Candida, the utilization of corticosteroids or different prescriptions that influence the safe framework, a debilitated insusceptible framework because of diabetes, pregnancy, or one more ailment and deficient drying of soggy skin. Warm, moist environments are ideal for the growth of Candida fungi. Because of this, the condition frequently affects skin folds. Additionally, candidiasis of the skin can occur in infants, particularly on the buttocks. Candida typically thrives in an environment created by a diaper. Candidiasis of the skin normally isn't infectious. In any case, individuals with debilitated resistant frameworks might foster the condition after contacting the skin of a tainted individual.

Candida is also more likely to cause severe infections in people who have weak immune systems.

Symptoms of candidiasis of the skin

The primary side effect of candidiasis of the skin is a rash. The rash frequently causes redness and serious tingling. The infection may occasionally result in cracked and swollen skin. Additionally, blisters and pustules may occur. The rash can appear anywhere on the body, but it is most likely to appear in the skin's folds. This remembers regions for the armpits, in the crotch, between the fingers, and under the bosoms. Candida can likewise cause contaminations in the nails, edges of the nails, and corners of the mouth. Different circumstances that might look like candidiasis of the skin include: ringworm, hives, herpes, diabetes-related skin conditions, contact, dermatitis, seborrheic dermatitis, dermatitis, and psoriasis.

An infection that causes white sores in the mouth, throat, esophagus, or tongue is called oral candidiasis (thrush). Thrush is a yeast-like fungal infection that can spread to your mouth, throat, and other body parts. You may develop spots (white, raised, resembling cottage cheese) on your tongue and cheeks if you have oral candidiasis. Thrush can immediately become bothered and cause mouth torment and redness. Thrush happens when there's an excess of Candida, a sort of organism. Oropharyngeal candidiasis is another name for thrush in the

throat or mouth. Thrush is treated by healthcare providers with antifungal medication. On the off chance that your insusceptible framework is solid, thrush is a minor issue that disappears a long time after you start treatment. Thrush can affect anyone, but some people are more likely to get it, like babies younger than one month, toddlers, adults over the age of 65, and people with weaker immune systems (whose symptoms are harder to control).

Causes thrush

Thrush can also affect adults. The majority of people have very little Candida fungus in their skin, digestive tract, and mouth. At the point when diseases, stress, or meds upset this equilibrium, the parasite outgrows control and causes thrush. Drugs that can make yeast thrive and cause disease incorporate Corticosteroids, Anti-toxins, and Contraception pills. Is the thrush infectious? Those who are at risk, such as those with weakened immune systems or who take certain medications, may contract thrush. It is uncommon for people with strong immune systems to contract thrush through kissing or other close contact. The majority of the time, thrush is not particularly contagious—that is, it does not spread from one person to another—but it is transmittable—that is, you can catch it through other means. Avoid coming into contact with another person's saliva (spit) if you are concerned about

contracting thrush from them. If you are near someone who has thrush, it is wise to wash your hands as frequently as possible.

Candida granuloma: A serious, persistent disease that objectives your skin, scalp, mouth, or fingernails. Obtrusive candidiasis (foundational candidiasis): A serious disease that happens all through your body, frequently in your circulatory system or on the layer coating of your heart or skull, because of a lack of safety.

Causes Of Candidiasis
1. Albicans coccus   Essential Offender: Candida albicans is the most well-known species liable for candidiasis. It thrives in warm, moist places like the mouth, digestive system, and genital area.
Pathogen opportunistic: Candida is normally controlled by our immune system. However, Candida can rapidly multiply and cause infections when certain conditions encourage its growth, such as a weaker immune system or changes in hormones.

2. Immunosuppression   Weakened Immune Systems: The immune system is compromised by HIV/AIDS, chemotherapy, and organ transplants. Accordingly, the body battles to control Candida's abundance. Susceptibility: Candida is more common

in mucosal areas—the oral cavity, throat, and genital regions—in people whose immune systems are suppressed.

3. Anti-toxins and Meds Disruption of Gut Flora: Taking antibiotics for an extended period alters the microbiota balance in the gut. Useful microscopic organisms are diminished, permitting Candida to prosper unrestrained.

Different Meds: Corticosteroids, immunosuppressants, and conception prevention pills can likewise disturb the stomach microbiome, establishing a climate helpful for Candida development.

4. Lifestyle and diet Sugar and Carbs: High sugar admission and refined starches give more than adequate fuel to Candida. Sugars feed the yeast, prompting excess.

Drinking too much alcohol: Drinking too much alcohol, especially in excess, weakens the immune system and affects gut health.

 Poor nutrition, chronic stress, and insufficient sleep all weaken the immune system, making people more likely to develop candidiasis.

5. Preexisting Medical Conditions Diabetes: Diabetes creates an ideal environment for Candida due to elevated blood sugar levels.

Obesity: Candidiasis is brought on by being overweight and the inflammation that comes with it.

Hormonal imbalances: The body's defenses against Candida are affected by pregnancy, hormonal therapies, and menstrual cycles. People are empowered to take preventative measures and seek timely treatment when they are aware of these causes. By tending to these elements, we can more readily oversee and forestall candidiasis.

Prevalence
Candidiasis influences different populations around the world:
Vaginal Candidiasis: Normal among ladies, with side effects like tingling, copying, and unusual release.
Oral Thrush: Frequently found in newborn children, the old, and immunocompromised people. It is characterized by white patches on the tongue and inner cheeks.
Cutaneous Candidiasis: Infections of the skin can occur in warm, moist areas like the groin, under the breasts, and folds of the skin. Foundational Candidiasis: Uncommon yet serious, influencing inner organs. It happens to people who are seriously ill or have a weak immune system.

Managing the Overgrowth of Yeast

 1. Personal satisfaction: Ongoing Effect: Candidiasis, when left untreated or undiscovered, can essentially lessen personal satisfaction. Imagine waking up each day with exhaustion, mental confusion, and physical discomfort. Work, relationships, and daily activities can all be impacted by these symptoms. Physical and Profound Cost: Stomach-related issues, skin issues, and mindset aggravations (like uneasiness and peevishness) become steady friends. Individuals can seek prompt intervention if they recognize these symptoms early.

2. Problems with misdiagnosis:

The Great Mimicker: Candidiasis frequently takes on the appearance of other illnesses. It is misdiagnosed because its symptoms overlap with those of other health conditions. Healthcare providers may focus on unrelated causes if they are unaware, delaying effective treatment.

Consideration in Differential Diagnosis: Patients and healthcare professionals alike can include candidiasis as a possible differential diagnosis by comprehending it. This ensures accurate management and a more thorough evaluation.

3. Comprehensive Methodology:

Beyond Medications: Antifungal drugs are necessary, but they are only one part of the solution. A holistic approach supports overall health and addresses the underlying causes.

 Way of life Adjustments: Dietary changes (lessening sugar and refined carbs), stress the board, and streamlining rest assume a critical part. This way of life changes establish a climate less helpful for Candida's development.

4. Long-Term Stability: Empowerment through Knowledge: When people are aware of candidiasis, they can take control of their health. They can embrace preventive measures, perceive early indications of repeat, and keep up with versatility. Maintainable Health: Long haul the executives includes regarding intense contaminations as well as forestalling future episodes. Combating candidiasis becomes a commitment for the rest of one's life.

Keep in mind that candidiasis is more than just a bother; it is also a health problem that needs to be solved. We open the way to vitality and well-being by deciphering its complexities.

Chapter 2. The Bacterium Candida

Candida albicans is a fungus that grows on your body naturally. Candida is yeast, a kind of growth, that that is commonly tracked down in limited quantities on your mouth, skin, and in your digestion tracts. The balance of Candida in your body is controlled by healthy bacteria in your microbiome. Candidiasis is a condition in which the yeast overgrows and becomes infected when it is out of balance. Candida albicans is the kind of yeast that lives in your body. If the balance of good bacteria and yeast is off, it can grow too much and become infected. An infection brought on by excessive yeast (Candida) growth is referred to as candidiasis. Thrush, diaper rash, and vaginal yeast infection are all common infections.

Contributing Factors to Candida Overgrowth
A few elements can disturb the sensitive harmony among Candida and solid microbes, prompting excess:

1. Antibiotics Mechanism: Although antibiotics are made to kill bad bacteria, they can also affect good bacteria in the gut. Candida can flourish when the equilibrium is disturbed.

Impact: Taking antibiotics for an extended time can cause dysbiosis, or a flora imbalance in the gut, which allows Candida albicans to grow.

Avoidance: Assuming you want anti-toxins, consider probiotic supplementation to keep up with stomach wellbeing.

2. Diet

Candida loves sugar and refined carbohydrates. An eating regimen high in refined sugars and basic carbs gives more than adequate fuel to its development. Influence: Exorbitant sugar utilization takes care of Candida, prompting excess.

Counteraction: Choose a fair eating regimen rich in whole grains, vegetables, and lean proteins. Reduce your intake of processed foods and sweets.

3. Drinking habits

Immune Suppression: Because alcohol weakens the immune system, your body will have a harder time controlling Candida.

Impact: Consuming alcohol regularly can break down the gut barrier and encourage Candida colonization.

Avoidance: Breaking point liquor admission and remain hydrated.

4. Debilitated Safe Framework

The immune system is compromised by HIV, diabetes, and other immunosuppressive conditions.

 Influence: Candida excess is more probable in people with debilitated resistance. Anticipation: Oversee basic ailments and focus on invulnerable help.

5. Pills for contraception

Changes in Hormones: Birth control pills affect the vaginal environment by altering hormone levels.

Effect: A favorable environment for Candida growth can be created by hormonal fluctuations.

Anticipation: If you're inclined to yeast contaminations, talk about elective preventative techniques with your medical care supplier.

6. High Feelings of anxiety

 Immunity and stress: Chronic stress weakens the immune system and disturbs the microbiome's equilibrium.

 Influence: Stress chemicals can change stomach greenery, inclining toward Candida.

 Prevention: Use techniques like meditation, exercise, and getting enough sleep to reduce stress.

How Candida Means for Various Body Frameworks

 Mouth and Throat (Thrush): Candida excess in the mouth prompts white, raised knocks on the tongue, internal cheeks, gums, tonsils, or throat. In severe cases, the infection may spread to the esophagus, resulting in pain or difficulty swallowing. The condition of oral thrush, also known as oral candidiasis (kan-dih-DIE-uh-sis), occurs when the fungus Candida albicans builds up on the lining of your mouth. Although Candida is a normal organism that lives in your mouth, it can sometimes grow too much and cause symptoms. Creamy white lesions are the result of oral thrush, usually on the inside of your cheeks or tongue. The roof of your mouth, your gums or tonsils, or the back of your throat may occasionally be affected by oral thrush. Even though oral thrush can affect anyone, it is more likely to affect babies and older adults who have a lower immune system, other people whose immune systems are suppressed or who have certain health conditions, or people who take certain medications. If you are healthy, oral thrush is a minor issue; however, if you have a weak immune system, the symptoms may be more severe and difficult to manage. Regularly, your invulnerable framework attempts to repulse unsafe attacking creatures, for example, infections, microscopic organisms, and growths, while keeping harmony among "great" and "terrible" microorganisms that ordinarily occupy your body. However, there are times when these protective mechanisms fail, increasing the number of candida fungi and the development of an oral thrush infection. Candida albicans is the most prevalent type of candida fungus.

A few variables, like a debilitated safe framework, can expand your gamble of oral thrush.

 Fatigue: Although it has not been directly demonstrated, nutritional deficiencies (such as magnesium) and a weakened immune system may be linked to fatigue in candidiasis patients. Fatigue is one of the most common symptoms of Candida. While there's no proof that Candida causes exhaustion, there are several manners by which it could add to it. In the first place, candidiasis is in many cases joined by dietary lacks, like vitamin B6, fundamental unsaturated fats, and magnesium. Fatigue has been linked to magnesium deficiency in particular. Second, Candida diseases usually happen when the resistant framework is debilitated. A low-working safe framework in itself might leave you feeling drained and exhausted. Long-term candidiasis of the gut may even be a potential cause of chronic fatigue syndrome, according to a 1995 study. However, more investigation is required.

Infections of the vagina: When Candida multiplies in the vagina, it causes discomfort and itching, which is known as vaginal yeast infection (candida vaginitis). Several conditions that can infect or irritate your vagina are referred to as vaginitis. Inflammation of both the vagina and the vulva, or external part of your genitals, is referred to as vulvovaginitis, which is a generic term for both conditions. Vaginal diseases can have a lot of various causes, and they're genuinely normal. According to the American College of Obstetricians and Gynecologists, vaginitis affects up to a third of women who have a vagina. These diseases can occur whenever, however, they're generally normal during your regenerative years, or your late youngsters to mid-40s. You can foster vaginal contamination without having penetrative sex, or some other kind of sex. To put it another way, a sexually transmitted infection (STI) and vaginitis are not the same thing. However, certain types of sexual activity may occasionally have something to do with the yeast infection.

Types of infections that can occur in the genital area Because many of the symptoms of a vaginal infection are the same, it can be hard to tell exactly what's going on. All things considered, each kind of contamination includes a couple of novel side effects:

Bacterial vaginosis (BV): BV frequently results in a thin discharge that is greenish, grayish-white, or yellow. This release can have a fish-like scent that will in general become more grounded after penetrative vaginal sex. You might not feel much itchiness.

Itching, burning, and tenderness in the vaginal and vulval areas are typical symptoms of yeast infections. Swelling in the labia or the folds of skin on the outside of your vagina can also be a sign of yeast infections. Any release will for the most part be white and uneven, with a surface that some say looks like curds.

Trichomoniasis: This infection typically causes a fish-like odor and itchy vagina. You might also notice swelling, irritation, and inflammation in your vulva in addition to a frothy, greenish-yellow discharge. Pain during vaginal sex, lower abdominal pain, and burning and pain during urination are additional signs of trichomoniasis.

Atrophic vaginitis: This isn't contamination, precisely, yet it can build your possibility of creating vaginal diseases and UTIs. You might experience symptoms of atrophic vaginitis that are similar to those of other infections, such as dryness, vaginal itching, burning, and changes in discharge.

Causes Vaginal Diseases

In simple terms, when something disturbs the normal balance of bacteria and yeast in your vagina, infections tend to occur. By type of infection, the most common causes of vaginal infections are as follows:

Bacterial contaminations: An excess of specific microbes normally found in your vagina can cause BV. While BV isn't viewed as an STI, sexual contact — including hand-to-genital, oral, and penetrative vaginal sex — can prompt microbes abundance and increment your possibilities of creating BV.

Yeast contaminations: Yeast diseases are normally brought about by a parasite called Candida albicans. Antibiotics, hormonal changes, a weak immune system, stress, and other factors can all reduce the number of antifungal bacteria in your vagina, resulting in excessive yeast growth. Symptoms of a yeast infection may result from this excessive growth.

Trichomoniasis: The protozoan parasite Trichomonas vaginalis causes this contamination. Having vaginal, oral, or anal sex without an internal or external condom is the most common way to contract trichomoniasis. However, there is evidence to suggest that you could contract it by sharing bathwater. Pools, damp towels or clothing, and damp toilet seats are other uncommon but possible transmission methods.

Vaginal decay: This condition for the most part creates after menopause, however it can likewise happen while you're nursing or whatever other time when you experience a drop in estrogen levels. Diminished chemical levels can cause vaginal diminishing and dryness, which can prompt vaginal aggravation.

Douching: It may seem like a good idea to clean your vagina by flushing it with a vinegar-water mixture, baking soda, iodine, or other antiseptic ingredients. However, the truth is that your vagina can remain clean on its own. This practice reduces the amount of good bacteria in your vagina, increasing the likelihood of infections. While it is acceptable to rinse your vulva and vagina with plain water, any other product or fragrance can kill healthy bacteria in your vagina and increase the likelihood of infection. Soap, body wash, and perfume: Washing your vagina with soap and body wash or spraying it with perfume can also disrupt its natural pH.

Spermicidal contraceptives: This strategy for anti-conception medication could come in gel, film, or suppository structure. You embed it straightforwardly into your vagina, where it disintegrates to kill sperm and forestall undesirable pregnancy. While spermicides function admirably for certain individuals, they can prompt vaginal disturbance and irritation, and they can make vaginal diseases more probable.

Tight-fitting or engineered clothing: Clothing and bottoms that can't "relax" can cause vaginal disturbance by catching dampness and forestalling wind current, which can make diseases more probable. Similar effects can result from wearing very tight bottoms or leaving wet bottoms on after a swim or workout.

Cleanser and cleanser: Have you noticed any symptoms as soon as you changed your laundry products? Scented cleansers and cleansers can likewise influence vaginal pH and add to yeast contaminations.

 Systemic Candidiasis is a rare but serious infection that affects the blood, bones, brain, and heart as well as the entire body. It as a rule happens in hospitalized people or those with debilitated resistance. A variety of yeast infections caused by

various species (types) of Candida are included in systemic
candidiasis. It is a serious infection that can spread to the blood,
heart, brain, eyes, bones, and other body parts. Ninety percent
of systemic candidiasis cases are caused by five distinct species
of Candida, out of more than 200 species. When Candida enters
the bloodstream (candidemia), this invasive yeast infection
takes the most common form. Fever and chills are symptoms of
candidemia and do not improve with antibiotic treatment. The
infected organ or system determines the symptoms of other
forms of systemic candidiasis. Fundamental candidiasis is the
most widely recognized contagious contamination among
hospitalized individuals in top-level salary nations, including
the US. Analysis can be troublesome, particularly when the
Candida isn't tracked down in the circulatory system.

Chapter 3. Symptoms And Signs

Signs and side effects of candidiasis fluctuate contingent on the area impacted. Although the majority of candida infections only cause minor complications like redness, itchiness, and discomfort, certain populations may experience severe or even fatal complications if they are not treated. Onychomycosis, a localized infection of the skin, fingernails, toenails, or mucosal membranes, such as the oral cavity and pharynx (thrush), esophagus, and the sex organs (vagina, penis, etc.), is the most common form of candidiasis in healthy people who are immune-competent. In healthy people, the gastrointestinal tract, urinary tract, and respiratory tract Candida infections in the esophagus are more common in immunocompromised people than in healthy people and have a greater chance of spreading throughout the body, leading to a much more serious condition known as candidemia. Side effects of esophageal candidiasis incorporate trouble gulping, agonizing gulping, stomach agony, sickness, and regurgitating.

Mouth: Disease in the mouth is described by white stains on the tongue, around the mouth, and in the throat. Additionally, irritation may occur, resulting in discomfort when swallowing. Thrush is normally found in babies. It isn't viewed as strange in newborn children except if it endures longer than half a month.

Genitals: A whitish or whitish-gray cottage cheese-like discharge and severe itching, burning, and irritation are common symptoms of vaginal or vulvar infection. Red skin around the head of the penis, swelling, irritation, itchiness, and soreness of the head of the penis, thick, lumpy discharge under the foreskin, an unpleasant odor, difficulty retracting the foreskin (phimosis), and pain when passing urine or during sex are all signs of balanitis thrush, an infection of the male genitalia.

Skin: Signs and side effects of candidiasis in the skin incorporate tingling, bothering, and abrading or broken skin.

Invasive Disease: In healthy people, anal itching, belching, bloating, indigestion, nausea, diarrhea, gas, intestinal cramps, vomiting, and gastric ulcers are typical symptoms of gastrointestinal candidiasis. Perianal candidiasis can cause butt-centric tingling; the sore can be red, papular, or ulcerative for all intents and purposes, and being a physically sent infection isn't thought of. Dysbiosis can result from abnormal candida growth in the intestines. While it isn't yet clear, this change might be the wellspring of side effects commonly depicted as crabby gut conditions and other gastrointestinal sicknesses.

Neurological side effects

Foundational candidiasis can influence the focal sensory system causing various neurological side effects, with a show like meningitis.

Acute Vs Chronic Infections

The body's presence of harmful microorganisms like bacteria, viruses, fungi, yeast, and parasites is the root cause of infections. These miniature creatures can increase and cause a disease, which can go from gentle to serious. Some infections might not have any symptoms at all, while others might have obvious symptoms like fever, pain, or inflammation. An infection can affect only one part of the body or spread throughout the body through the blood or lymphatic system. It's essential to take note that not all microorganisms present in the body are viewed as contaminations, as some, for example, the microscopic organisms present in the mouth and digestion tracts, are viewed as typical and gainful. Good hygiene, such as washing your hands frequently and avoiding close contact with sick people, is essential for infection prevention.

What exactly is an acute illness?

A type of infection known as an acute infection typically manifests quickly and only lasts for a short time. It typically has a duration of less than six months. Notwithstanding, late examination proposes that intense contaminations can significantly affect the host's well-being, possibly expanding the gamble of persistent infections like immune system illnesses, sensitivities, and ongoing weariness condition. The common cold, the flu, acute appendicitis, acute respiratory tract infections, acute kidney infections, and acute bladder infections are all examples of acute infections. Antibiotics or other medications are typically used to treat these kinds of infections, assisting in the fight against the invading microorganisms and relieving symptoms.

What is an Ongoing Contamination?

A type of infection known as a chronic infection is one that lasts for a significant amount of time—typically longer than six months. The body's immune system is unable to fully respond to and eliminate the infecting microorganisms in contrast to acute infections, allowing them to continue to thrive and cause inflammation. This can prompt an assortment of medical issues, including healthful inadequacies, weight on the adrenal organs, and a debilitated invulnerable framework. Lyme disease, mold toxicity, Hepatitis C, HIV/AIDS, Epstein-Barr Virus, HPV,

COVID-19, and chronic fatigue syndrome (CFS) are all examples of chronic infections. It may be necessary to manage symptoms and improve overall health with a combination of medications and lifestyle modifications for these kinds of infections, which can be challenging to diagnose and treat. If you think you might have a chronic infection, it's important to see a doctor right away because early diagnosis and treatment can help keep serious problems from happening.

How are diseases treated?

Diseases can be treated in different ways depending upon the particular kind of contamination and the seriousness of the side effects. One normal treatment for diseases is the utilization of anti-infection agents, which can assist with killing the tainting miniature organic entities. Nonetheless, anti-microbials may not be viable in treating a wide range of contaminations, and they can likewise make side impacts. Additionally, antibiotic overuse may result in antibiotic resistance, making it more challenging to treat subsequent infections.

Effects on mental well-being

Perhaps the earliest specialist to distribute discoveries about the association between Candida and gloom is Dr. Orian Support. His persuasive work has been mentioned in some books and has assisted numerous patients thus far. Interestingly, the psychiatric community, which had just begun to observe the effects of MAO inhibitors at the time, did not pay much attention to his discovery in 1981. While these and other current antidepressants remain significant devices for treating mental patients, studies have exhibited that their adequacy rate is something like 20-30 percent (Kroenke, Hansen). We lack sufficient comprehension of the extensive range of mental disorders that affect millions of people. We should take no shortcuts in this regard. Particularly assuming that stone has previously been displayed to give accommodating data. Dr. Truss hypothesized that while some people only experience Candida as a nuisance, others suffer from chronic illness, including mental illness. Although it is not necessary to have HIV or leukemia to suffer, those with compromised immune systems are particularly vulnerable. At the Huxley conference (1981), he introduced 6 contextual investigations he accepted to include the alleged Candida disorder that he found. Multiple courses of antibiotics or other immunosuppressants had been administered to each individual. The majority of these people were female. Almost always, depression was one of many ambiguous symptoms. Loss of memory, trouble concentrating, aversion to synthetics, and different side effects were likewise noted. Dr. Truss began incorporating antifungal therapy into treatment for patients with persistent mental illness.

Surprisingly, all of the people responded to the treatment, and their depression symptoms subsided.

Nystatin, an antifungal medication, was found to be significantly more effective than placebo in reducing depression symptoms in polysymptomatic patients in a 2001 double-blind placebo-controlled study led by Heiko Santelmann. The study's authors noted that people with mental complaints saw some of the most significant improvements. While nystatin isn't intended for Candida, a convincing report shows yeast can influence emotional wellness. Dr. Truss noted that testing for Candida is difficult because nearly everyone has been exposed to the organism. Deciding how much every individual endures depends on a bunch of unclear side effects that frequently end with the patient being named as psychosomatic or mental. Fortunately, we now have better methods for identifying Candida and a deeper comprehension of the mechanism that may be triggering symptoms. Pathogens' virulence-enhancing mechanisms have been identified thanks to genetic coding. In the case of Candida albicans, a particular gene that encodes Immunogenic Alcohol Dehydrogenase was identified in 1994 (Bertram). This compound produces acetyl aldehyde from glucose or ethanol (Gainza-Cirauqui). This acetyl aldehyde establishes a climate that isn't helpful for most microorganisms, successfully diminishing the contest. In people, acetyl aldehyde is a cancer-causing compound that effectively passes the blood-cerebrum boundary where it obstructs neurotransmission (Correa). Natural killer cell cytotoxicity decreases when depression and acetyl aldehyde are present (Irwin). A brief bout of depression may increase the likelihood of developing a chronic condition because nearly everyone has Candida in their body. Candida testing has always relied on a sensitive yeast culture. This test has the advantage of being able to identify the precise yeast species, allowing for the implementation of the appropriate treatment. This approach has the drawback of being well-known for generating false negatives (Maaroufi). Metabolites of yeast distinguished in The Incomparable Fields Research Center Natural Acids Test are a truly dependable technique for identifying Candida excess (Shaw). This test cannot identify the exact organism, but this is of little consequence. The most prevalent yeast species, Candida albicans, is effectively eradicated by the majority of prescription antifungals (Shaw). Furnished with the right data, the most recent in analytic testing, and reasonable treatment choices, mental and essential considerations doctors can practice various choices for patients with side effects of melancholy and other psychological well-being problems. Numerous doctors are turning to comprehensive testing for yeast (and other pathogens) to find solutions to psychiatric diseases that are as complex as the patients themselves. It makes sense to inquire as to whether this is related to Candida or another pathogen in a patient who presents with a recent onset of chronic depression in the absence of major trauma. Doing so could save your patient's life—or at least the life they used to have!

Chapter 4: Diagnostic Techniques

Lab tests: Blood, stool, and pee examination
There are a few different tests that can be used to identify Candida overgrowth if you suspect it. These include: Candida testing can be done in four different ways:

1. Stool Test: This test looks at a sample of stool to see if there is too much Candida in the gut. The universally adored: crap! Can Candida be found with a stool test? It absolutely can! A simple and enlightening technique to lead in the protection of your own home, a Floré Stomach Wellbeing test can not just let you know if you have a Candida excess but can likewise highlight experiences on over 23,000+ organisms in the stomach, which incorporate growth, microorganisms, yeast, infections and parasites.

Step 1: A Gut Health Test Kit is sent directly to you by us. When you gather your example and send it back to us, our committed group of Floré Researchers extricate your DNA from your example and dissect your microbiome, opening the mysteries of your stomach!

Step 2: Your results come with a custom report and a customized blend of synbiotics—prebiotics and probiotics based on your specific needs—to help align potential gut imbalances and maintain a healthy digestive system. This is more than just a Candida test.

Stage 3: You have the choice to talk with a Floré Researcher who will walk you through your stomach well-being report.

Indications of Candida in your stool

There are no obvious signs or symptoms in your sample, in case you feel tempted to examine it yourself. However, the color of your poop can tell a lot! Except for the potential bothersome diarrhea symptom we mentioned earlier, the color and texture of your stool may not be related to Candida overgrowth. If your poop is green, brown, or has a yellowish hue, do you know which ones aren't cause for concern?

2. Candida Blood Test - checks for the presence of Candida antibodies in the circulation system, which can be an indication of fundamental Candida excess. This test requires an outing to your PCP. A blood test looks at your antibodies, and a blood test for Candida overgrowth specifically looks for specific markers like a specific carbohydrate that is embedded in the cells of Candida species. One non-culture-based technique checks for the presence of mannan antigen and against mannan antibodies in the conclusion of obtrusive candidiasis. Because high antibody levels can indicate causes other than a current Candida overgrowth or that your immune system has been triggered into producing antibodies to fight normal Candida levels, there are some questions regarding the accuracy of the test. This kind of test may indicate that a person has an imbalance in the past for some people, but it does not help determine the source of the imbalance or whether it is still present.

3. Pee Candida Test - dissects a pee test to check for the presence of Candida excess in the kidneys, bladder, or urinary plot. Organic acid tests, which are also used to test urine, measure the levels of organic compounds in the urine that are made by the body as part of several important biochemical pathways. To put it another way, this test looks for yeast and bacteria that would suggest an overgrowth of Candida. The disadvantage is that while it might demonstrate an excess, it can't let you know where it very well may be happening (skin, stomach, mouth, vaginal channel, and so forth).

4. Spit Candida Test - checks for the presence of Candida abundance in the mouth. This sort of Candida test is finished to pinpoint Candida in the mouth, otherwise known as oral thrush. A specialist might take a spit test to be shipped off to a lab for assessment. Be that as it may, more often than not, they'll have the option to tell by simply taking a gander at your mouth (for example your tongue might have a white or yellowish variety to it and would be red and enlarged).

Tests specific to Candida

Patients often think of candida as the first thing that's wrong in their gut. It frequently involves bacterial overgrowths, enzyme dysfunction that results in food intolerances, and potential fungal overgrowths. However, the more functional testing I perform, the more I realize that infections and overgrowths of fungi and molds may be the primary cause of persistent digestive symptoms. For candida overgrowths, we are looking at three different testing options today.

1. Candidiasis (Yeast Infections) in the Vagina: A small amount of vaginal discharge is typically taken by healthcare providers to diagnose vaginal candidiasis. They look at the example under a magnifying lens in the clinical office or send it to a lab for a parasitic culture. However, a positive fungal culture does not necessarily imply that Candida is causing symptoms; some women may have Candida in their genital area without experiencing any symptoms.

2. Mouth or Throat Candidiasis (Thrush): By simply looking inside, healthcare providers can typically identify candidiasis in the mouth or throat. In some cases, they take a little example from the mouth or throat, which is shipped off to a research center for testing (generally analyzed under a magnifying lens).

 3. Candidiasis of the Throat: An endoscopy is used by healthcare professionals to diagnose candidiasis in the esophagus. An endoscopy is a procedure in which a tube with a camera and a light is passed down the throat to examine the digestive system. Without an endoscopy to see if symptoms improve, antifungal medication may be prescribed in some instances1.

4. Intrusive Candidiasis: Blood culture is the primary method for diagnosing invasive candidiasis, which affects internal organs and causes infections in the bloodstream (candidemia). More up-to-date culture-free indicative strategies are promising but not yet broadly utilized. Although it is not particularly Candida-specific, the Beta-D-glucan assay is approved as an adjunctive diagnostic tool. Keep in mind that prompt treatment and testing can prevent serious infections. Consult your healthcare provider for the appropriate evaluation and treatment of candidiasis symptoms.

 Tests specific to Candida
1. Culture of fungi:
 - Objective: To find out if any species of Candida are present.

- The Process - A sample, such as blood, throat swab, or vaginal discharge, is taken.
- The example is refined on an extraordinary medium in the research center.   - The growth of Candida is observed and determined.
- Restrictions -It's possible that some Candida species won't thrive in culture.
- Bogus negatives can happen if the yeast is available however doesn't develop under unambiguous circumstances.

2. Assay for Beta-D-Glucan

- Objective: To find fungal infections like Candida.
- Method: - Measures the degree of beta-D-glucan (a contagious cell wall part) in blood.
- A fungal infection is suggested by elevated levels.
- Impediments: - Not limited to Candida; beta-D-glucan levels can be raised by other fungi as well.
- Misleading upsides can happen (e.g., because of bacterial tainting).

3. The PCR (polymerase chain reaction)

- Objective: To find DNA from Candida.
- Methodology: - Enhances particular segments of the Candida DNA.
- Distinguishes even limited quantities of Candida.
- Limits: - Requires expertise and specialized equipment.
- Misleading up-sides/negatives can happen.

4. Tests for Detecting Antigens

- Reason: To recognize Candida antigens (proteins).
 - Examples: -Candida Mannan Antigen: Recognizes mannans (Candida cell wall parts) in blood
-Candida Albicans Antibody Test: This test looks for antibodies to Candida.
 - Constraints: - Responsiveness and particularity change.   - False outcomes are possible.

5. Biopsy and histology

-Reason: To look at tissue tests.
 -Method: Tissue biopsy (e.g., from the throat, skin) is taken.
 Candida invasion is revealed by microscopic examination.
 Limitations: -Intrusive technique.
may overlook infections at the surface.

Differential diagnosis with other conditions

Separating Candida diseases from different circumstances can be trying because of covering side effects. Here are a few central issues to consider for a differential conclusion:

1. Vaginosis Bacterial (BV) Symptoms: A thin, grayish-white, fishy-smelling discharge.

Analysis: Amsel measures or Gram stain.

Key Contrasts: BV commonly misses the mark on extraordinary tingling and thick, white release found in Candida infections.

2. Trichomoniasis

Side effects: Foamy, yellow-green release with serious areas of strength, tingling, and inconvenience during peeing.
Microscopic examination or nucleic acid amplification tests (NAATs) are used for diagnosis.
 Important distinctions: Trichomoniasis typically presents with a frothy discharge and a stronger odor than Candida.

3. Dermatitis (Contact or Atopic)

Side effects: Red, bothersome, and aroused skin, once in a while with rankles. Finding: Clinical assessment and patient history.
Key Contrasts: Dermatitis is normally connected with outside aggravations or allergens and misses the mark on release regular of Candida.

4. Psoriasis

Skin patches that are red and covered in silvery scales are the signs. Clinical examination and biopsy are used to diagnose.
Important distinctions: Psoriasis lesions are more distinct and scaly than Candida3's erythematous patches.

5. Tinea (Ringworm): Infections Red, ring-shaped, scaly patches with a clear center are the symptoms. KOH test or fungal culture for diagnosis Key Contrasts: Fungus diseases have a trademark ring shape and are brought about by dermatophytes, not yeast.

6. Viruses and Infections

Side effects: Redness, expansion, torment, and at times discharge.

Conclusion: Culture and awareness tests. Important distinctions: Bacterial infections typically manifest as more localized pain and pus production1.

7. Other Intertrigo Types Red, inflamed skin in body folds are the symptoms. Clinical examination is used for diagnosis. Key Contrasts: Intertrigo can be brought about by microorganisms, parasites, or aggravations, and may not necessarily in all cases include Candida. Demonstrative Methodology Clinical Assessment: Evaluate side effects and actual signs.

Utilizing microscopy and culture, locate the causing organism. Consider risk factors and previous infections in the patient's history. An exact conclusion is critical for compelling treatment.

Chapter 5: Lifestyle Modifications

If you figure you might have a yeast disease, you ought to initially converse with your clinical supplier. Notwithstanding, a few food sources and dietary changes may likewise help. To combat Candida infections, here are five diet suggestions.

1. Coconut oil

Microscopic fungi known as Candida yeasts can be found in the skin, mouth, or gut. They are usually not harmful, but when your body's defenses are weak, they can cause infections. Some plants produce compounds that are harmful to fungi and have defenses against yeasts and other fungi. Saturated fatty acid lauric acid, which has been extensively studied for its antimicrobial and antifungal properties, is a good example. Lauric acid makes up nearly half of coconut oil. Because of this, it is one of the richest sources of this compound, which is rarely found in large quantities in food. Studies conducted in a test tube indicate that lauric acid is extremely effective against

Candida yeast. All things considered, coconut oil might make a comparative impact. As a result, oil pulling, or using coconut oil as a mouthwash, may help prevent thrush and Candida infections in the mouth. Remember that human studies are required to verify these benefits.

2. A low-sugar diet

When sugar is readily available, yeasts grow at a faster rate. Candida infections are more likely to occur in people who have high levels of sugar in their blood. In one study, mice with compromised immune systems and digestive systems saw an increase in Candida growth as a result of sugar. In a human study, rinsing the mouth with dissolved sugar was associated with an increase in infections and yeast counts. A different human study, on the other hand, found that a diet high in sugar did not affect Candida growth in the mouth or digestive system. However, there is a need for additional human studies. Regardless of whether a low-sugar diet may not generally be compelling against yeasts, wiping out added sugar from your eating regimen will work on your well-being in numerous alternate ways.

3. Garlic

Another food made of plants with strong antifungal properties is garlic. Allicin, a substance produced when fresh garlic is crushed or damaged, plays a role in this. Allicin appears to be slightly less effective than fluconazole, an antifungal medication, in combating Candida yeasts in mice when administered in large doses. Garlic extract may also make it harder for yeasts to attach to the cells in your mouth, according to research done in a test tube. However, whereas the majority of studies use high doses, garlic only contains trace amounts of allicin. One 14-day concentrate on ladies found that taking garlic supplements in some cases didn't influence vaginal yeast contaminations. In general, there is a need for additional clinical trials to determine whether eating garlic has any therapeutic value for humans. Nonetheless, adding garlic to food is safe and healthy. It could likewise function admirably close to traditional Candida medicines. Remember that involving crude garlic in touchy regions, like your mouth, can be hurtful and cause extreme compound consume

4. Curcumin

Curcumin is one of the dynamic parts of turmeric, a well-known Indian zest. Curcumin has been shown to inhibit the growth of Candida yeasts or kill them in test tubes. Curcumin may hinder yeasts' ability to attach to HIV-infected mouth cells, according to another study. The antifungal drug fluconazole was found to be less effective than curcumin. In any case, reviews are restricted to test tubes. It's hazy whether curcumin supplements have impacts on people.

Food To Stay away from

Added Sugars: Since Candida thrives on sugar, it's important to cut back on refined sugars and sugary snacks.

Handled Food varieties frequently contain additives and added substances that can upset stomach well-being. Whole grains and complex carbohydrates are better options than foods with a high glycemic index.

Liquor: Liquor can debilitate the insusceptible framework and advance candida development.

2. Healthy Gut Balance

1. Probiotics

When consumed, probiotics are live microorganisms, typically yeast or bacteria, that benefit the body's health. Their function is to promote the growth of beneficial bacteria, which aids in the maintenance of a balanced flora in the gut. Examples include yogurt, which contains live cultures like Bifidobacterium and Lactobacillus.

Kefir: A matured milk-savor-rich probiotic.

Kimchi: A Korean dish produced using matured vegetables.

Sauerkraut: Matured cabbage.

Enhanced immune function, improved digestion, and possibly relief from diarrhea and irritable bowel syndrome (IBS) are some of the advantages.

2. Prebiotics

Prebiotics are fibers that probiotics can't digest and use as food.
 Function: They give the good bacteria in your gut the food they need to grow and thrive.   For instance, onions contain a lot of inulin, a prebiotic fiber.
 Bananas: Particularly ready bananas contain safe starch, a prebiotic.
Inulin-rich asparagus supports gut health.
Inulin can also be found in garlic.
Important: Prebiotics support overall health and support a balanced microbiome.

3. Hydration

 Remaining hydrated is fundamental for ideal stomach capability.
Function: Consuming sufficient water aids in digestion, nutrient absorption, and waste elimination.
 Water: Go for the gold 8 cups (64 ounces) of water every day.
Herbal Teas: Teas containing chamomile, ginger, and peppermint can also help you stay hydrated.
Keep away from Exorbitant Caffeine and Liquor: These can dry out you.

3. Sleep hygiene and stress reduction Stress Decrease:

Persistent pressure debilitates the insusceptible framework, exacerbating candidiasis. Take up yoga, mindfulness, or hobbies.

Quality Rest: Focus on rest — hold back nothing hours daily. Sleep is good for your immune system and overall health. Keep in mind, that these way of life alterations supplement clinical treatment. Always seek individual guidance from a healthcare professional.

Chapter 6: Medical Treatments

In general, antifungal medications can either kill fungal cells directly or prevent fungal cells from growing and flourishing. But how do they accomplish this? To combat a fungal infection without causing damage to your body's cells, antifungal medications target structures or functions that are required in fungal cells but not in human cells. Two designs that are ordinarily focused on are the parasitic cell film and the contagious cell wall. The fungal cell is safeguarded by these two structures. The fungal cell may rupture and die when either one is compromised. While most fungal infections can be treated easily, some can be very serious. See your primary care physician if a contagious disease doesn't disappear with OTC treatment or on the other hand on the off chance that you suspect you have a more serious parasitic contamination. There are numerous antifungal medications. They can be administered orally, topically, or intravenously. The dosage of an antifungal medication is determined by many factors the drug itself, the type of infection, and its severity. The chemical structure and mechanism of action of antifungal medications are used to classify them. We'll go over the various antifungal medications and some examples of the infections they treat below.

Azoles

Some of the most widely used antifungals are azoles. They slow down a chemical that is significant for making the parasitic cell film. The cell membrane becomes unstable and susceptible to leakage as a result, eventually resulting in cell death. Imidazoles and triazoles are the two subgroups of azole antifungals. The conditions that imidazole antifungals treat include:

Candida infections of the skin and mucous membranes, blastomycosis, and histoplasmosis can all be treated with ketoconazole.

Infections of the skin and mucous membranes with clotrimazole Miconazole: skin and mucous film contaminations Triazoles are used to treat the following conditions:

Fluconazole: Cryptococcosis and Candida infections, including those that are invasive, systemic, and mucosal. Aspergillosis, blastomycosis, histoplasmosis, mucosal Candida infections, off-label coccidioidomycosis, and onychomycosis are all treated with itraconazole.

Posaconazole: off-label treatment for aspergillosis, mucosal, and invasive Candida infections

Voriconazole: aspergillosis, invasive or mucosal Candida infections, and Fusarium species infections
Isavuconazole: aspergillosis and mucormycosis Polyenes
Polyenes kill fungal cells by making the wall of the fungal cell more porous, making it more likely to burst.

Antifungals made of polyene include:
Amphotericin B: Off-label treatments for aspergillosis, blastomycosis, cryptococcosis, histoplasmosis, mucosal or invasive Candida infections, and coccidioidomycosis are available in a variety of formulations.
Nystatin is used to treat mouth and skin Candida infections.
Allylamines: Allylamines, like azole antifungals, stop working with an enzyme that makes the fungal cell membrane. Terbinafine, which is frequently used to treat skin fungal infections, is an example of an allylamine.
Echinocandins: Echinocandins are an upcoming class of antifungal medication. They prevent an enzyme from producing the fungal cell wall.
Echinocandins are, for instance: Anidulafungin: mucosal and intrusive Candida diseases Caspofungin: aspergillosis, mucosal and invasive Candida infections Micafungin: mucosal and

obtrusive Candida diseases there are additionally a few different kinds of antifungal drugs. These have mechanisms that are not the same as the ones we talked about above. Flucytosine is an antifungal that keeps the contagious cell from making nucleic acids and proteins. As a result, the cell is unable to expand and flourish. Systemic infections caused by either the Candida or Cryptococcus species can be treated with flucytosine. Griseofulvin inhibits the fungal cell's ability to divide and produce more cells. Skin, hair, and nail infections can all be treated with it.

Managing Infections That Recur

Your safe framework incorporates organs, lymph hubs, bone marrow, white platelets, protein, and different chemicals. Its responsibility is to avert microorganisms, organisms, parasites, and infections that can make you debilitated. However, there are times when your immune system is unable to effectively treat or prevent an illness or infection. Here's what you need to know if you keep getting sick or notice that you get one infection after another.

Symptoms of Recurring Infections

Repeat infections can sometimes be obvious. For instance, if you experience persistent urinary tract infections (UTIs), you are aware that your body is having difficulty fighting the infection. However, repeat infections may not always be obvious. If you have had any of the following: a cold or flu that goes away for a week or two before coming back. Multiple episodes of the painful rash known as shingles, which is brought on by the varicella-zoster virus, which is also responsible for chickenpox.

The chickenpox virus remains in your body after infection. Because your immune system is weaker, shingles can cause rashes in areas of your body where the virus is active. Repetitive pneumonia: This occurs when you have recovered from a serious lower respiratory infection known as pneumonia but then contract it again more than a month later.

Recurring Yeast Or Fungal Infections

If a prescription assisted you with disposing of vaginal yeast contaminations or parasitic diseases in your nails or feet, yet they returned a little while or months after the fact, your safe framework presumably isn't cleaning the disease off of your framework.

Reasons for Recurring Infections

Recurring infections can result from several factors, including: inadequate sleep: Your immune system fights infection and inflammation by releasing proteins called cytokines while you sleep. Your body will produce fewer cells and antibodies that fight infections if you don't get enough sleep or if the sleep you get isn't good enough. That increases your risk of contracting a virus. Additionally, it makes it more difficult for you to recover from illness. Smoking: Smoking weakens your immune system. It likewise makes changes to your lungs and aviation routes that make it more probable for you to become ill, and for that infection to be more serious.

Abuse of alcohol: Drinking too much can make your defenses less effective. There may be fewer immune cells in your system, and their effectiveness may suffer. Your immune system can be temporarily weakened by even a single binge. Repetitive infections can result from not washing your hands after using the bathroom or before touching your mouth and nose. This is especially true if you frequently get the flu or a cold. It may appear as though you are infected with the same virus, but different viruses could be at work. This is why it's so important to wash your hands several times a day with soap and water for at least 20 seconds, especially before eating or touching your face.

Factors inherited: A genetic predisposition may be the cause of some repeat infections, such as pneumonia and bladder infections. That is a genetic predisposition to contract more infections than the majority of people.

Underlying issues: Rehash diseases can likewise occur because of how your body is assembled. An abnormally shaped urinary tract, for instance, can make you more susceptible to infection.

Antibiotics: Taking antibiotics can make bacteria more resistant to them, especially if they are used too much or in the wrong way.

Diabetes can make things like yeast infections in the genital area more likely. This is because yeast can more easily bind to your vaginal cells when your blood sugar is high. Your body will change in other ways as a result of high blood sugar. For instance, it eases back your bloodstream and holds your nerves back from filling in also as they can. That can make it more likely for you to get the same infection again, especially in your feet and other places. autoimmune and immunodeficiency disorders, which doctors may refer to as such. There are more than 300 resistant problems. B-cell and T-cell deficiencies are two of the most prevalent: In autoimmune disorders, your body mistakenly attacks its tissues. Your body's ability to fight infection is hampered as a result. Rheumatoid arthritis and type 1 diabetes are two examples of common autoimmune disorders. Various myeloma: This is a kind of malignant growth that influences the plasma cells of your bone marrow. Your body uses antibodies produced by plasma cells to fight infections. Your body makes abnormal plasma cells when you have multiple myeloma, making it hard for your body to fight infection.

Chapter 7: Healthful Gut and Candida

A biome is a distinct ecosystem that is defined by its inhabitants and environment. A miniature biome containing trillions of microscopic organisms in your gut, which is located inside your intestines. Over a thousand species of bacteria, viruses, fungi, and parasites are among these microorganisms. The microbiome in your gut is unique to you. During vaginal delivery or breastfeeding (chestfeeding), infants inherit their first gut microbes. Your diet and other exposures to the environment later bring in new microbes to your biome. Your gut microbiota may also be diminished by some of these exposures. The majority of the microorganisms that live in our intestines interact symbiotically with us, their hosts. This indicates that the relationship benefits both of us. We provide them with food and a place to sleep, and they perform vital bodily functions. These beneficial microbes also aid in controlling potentially harmful ones. Your gut microbiome is like a diverse native garden that you rely on for healthy foods and medications. You also thrive when your garden is healthy and flourishing. However, if the soil is depleted or polluted, or if beneficial plants are being overrun by pests or weeds, it can disrupt your ecosystem as a whole.

Function

Your gut microbiome supports numerous body functions and interacts with numerous body systems. It is so active in your body that some doctors and other medical professionals have said it's like an organ. We are still learning about some of these interactions, while others are well-known.

Digestive System

Certain dietary fibers and complex carbohydrates that you are unable to break down on your own are broken down by bacteria in your gut. Byproducts include the production of short-chain fatty acids, an important nutrient. In addition, they supply the enzymes needed to make certain vitamins, such as vitamins B1, B9, B12, and K. Although they may appear to be insignificant nutrients, micronutrient deficiencies can have a significant impact on your health. (See deficiencies in folate, vitamin K, and vitamin B12, respectively.) Particularly, short-chain fatty acids nourish the cells that line your gut and contribute to the overall health of your gut environment. Your intestines' bile is also metabolized by gut bacteria. To assist you in digesting fats, your liver sends bile to your small intestine. Bacteria and their

enzymes help break it down after that so that your liver can re-
absorb and recycle the bile acids. Enterohepatic circulation
refers to this. Your body wouldn't be able to recycle bile acids
and your liver wouldn't have enough to make new bile if this
process stopped working. You wouldn't get the bile your body
needs to digest and absorb fats. Additionally, residual
cholesterol, which is a component of bile, would accumulate in
your blood.

System of defense

Your immune system can learn to distinguish between
beneficial and pathogenic microbes in your gut thanks to the
assistance of beneficial microbes. Your gut is the largest organ
of your immune system and houses up to 80% of your immune
cells. These cells contribute to the daily elimination of
numerous pathogens. Additionally, beneficial gut microbes
compete directly with undesirable ones for nutrients and real
estate, preventing them from taking up too much space. A
weakened gut microbiome is directly linked to some of the
chronic bacterial infections that can affect your GI tract, such as
C. difficile and H. pylori. The beneficial gut bacteria's
byproducts, short-chain fatty acids, have significant advantages
for your immune system. They keep the bacteria and toxins
inside from getting into your bloodstream by maintaining your
gut barrier. They also have gut-friendly anti-inflammatory

properties. Your immune system is responsible for inflammation, but it can malfunction and become hyperreactive.

Chronic inflammation may play a role in numerous other diseases, including cancer, and is a feature of autoimmune disease. These kinds of inflammatory responses appear to be suppressed by short-chain fatty acids. vascular system Through the gut-brain axis, a network of nerves, neurons, and neurotransmitters that runs through your GI tract, gut microbes can affect your nervous system. Neurotransmitters like serotonin, which send chemical signals to your brain, are produced or stimulated by certain bacteria. Your nervous system may also be affected by bacterial products. While bacterial toxins have the potential to harm nerves, short-chain fatty acids have beneficial effects. The gut microbiome may play a role in a variety of neurological, behavioral, nerve pain, and mood disorders, according to ongoing research.

System of hormones

Endocrine cells in your gut lining interact with gut microbes and their products as well. Your gut is the largest organ of your endocrine system thanks to these cells, also known as enteroendocrine cells. They release hormones that control metabolism-related factors like blood sugar, hunger, and satiety. The metabolic syndrome, which includes obesity, insulin resistance, type 2 diabetes, and liver fat storage are still areas of

interest for researchers. Although the specific relationship between these conditions and certain gut microbiota is still unclear, there is some connection.

Strategies for Getting Your Gut Back in Shape
In our intestines, there are approximately 100 trillion microbes. Our gut flora, also known as our gut microbiome, is a community of living bacteria, viruses, yeasts, and other microbes. Most people used to think of bacteria, or "germs," as enemies that needed to be killed until recently. However, as scientists learn more about our gut flora, we are slowly realizing how important it is to take care of it. We are aware that the production of vitamins and the prevention of infections by our microbiome contribute to our health. It can even assist us in drug activation. The disease can result from anything that upsets the balance of microbes in our gut. Modern life wreaks havoc on our gut bugs, which is unfortunate. Antibiotics kill both good and bad bacteria, and they don't like processed foods like we do. In contrast to the environment in which our microbiomes co-evolved with us, we now live sanitized, sedentary indoor lives and are afraid of dirt. The outcome? lack of variety. This indicates that even though we all have roughly the same total number of microbes in our guts, many of us have

fewer species. That's not ideal because each species has a distinct

characteristics and functions linked to distinct aspects of human health.

14 Quick Ways Ao Restore A Healthy Gut Microbiome
A diet high in nutrients and fiber is the most effective strategy for restoring gut harmony. The good news is that your next meal can start changing the flora in your gut. According to research, the communities of our gut bacteria begin to shift almost immediately when we alter our diets. However, scientists have also discovered that when antibiotics are administered repeatedly and cause significant gut damage, some bacterial communities vanish and are unlikely to return. Because it is almost impossible to define a healthy microbiome, it is difficult to determine whether you have restored it. The flora in our guts varies greatly across the globe and our lifespans. Bifidobacteria, for instance, typically occupy the majority of a baby's gut until they begin eating solid foods. When compared to an adult microbiome, this lack of diversity is precisely what they require to get the most out of milk! Diversity is crucial, as research has repeatedly demonstrated. You are more likely to be healthy if you have more families of bacteria in your gut. There are stool tests that can give a window into your stomach. These show the levels of

inflammation, certain parasites, yeasts, and families of bacteria
that scientists believe are beneficial or harmful to your health.

Therefore, although you cannot "restore" your gut microbiome,
you can improve it. How to do it:

1. Fill your plate with foods high in polyphenols.
Polyphenols are substances in plant foods that our small
intestines do not fully absorb. This indicates that they transform
into substances with prebiotic, anti-inflammatory, anti-
oxidative, anti-carcinogenic, and anti-microbial properties after
being consumed by the microbes in our colon.

2. Establish a routine for sleeping; The microbiome research
of the last five years has demonstrated that the microbial
residents of our gut have their sleep schedules. One study found
that people who had experienced jet lag had a higher number of
bacteria in their guts that were linked to obesity and metabolic
disease. A more varied gut microbiome has been shown to
improve sleep quality in other studies.

3. Avoid the common Western diet; The evidence that a
modern diet high in processed foods, sugar, and low in fiber is
bad for our health is getting stronger by the day. "an
evolutionarily unique selection ground for microbes that can
promote diverse forms of inflammatory disease," according to a
recent study. This indicates that the essential good bacteria in

our guts aren't so keen on our inadequate diets, whereas the harmful ones appear to enjoy it.

4. Get some, but not too much, exercise; Over the past ten years, the science of this has accelerated. We now know that

exercise directly affects the bacteria in our gut, which in turn improves our insulin resistance, cardiorespiratory fitness, and tissue metabolism. However, excessive exercise causes our bodies to perceive it as a threat, which triggers the stress response and reduces the diversity of our gut flora.

 5. Double your intake of fiber; We cannot extract any nutrients from fiber, unlike horses, elephants, or cows, so it is not even food for us. However, our gut bacteria thrive on it. The evidence for the advantages of a diet high in fiber is overwhelming. One study found that a low-fiber diet can significantly reduce the diversity of our gut flora, increasing the risk of Crohn's disease, ulcerative colitis liver disease, colorectal cancer, metabolic syndrome, and obesity-related diseases.

6. Eliminate sugar from your diet; Your microbiome uses added sugar like rocket fuel. That sounds like a good thing, but it seems to encourage some families of bacteria to "take over," crowd out others, and send a healthy gut into dysbiosis, which is not good. In one study, mice fed a diet high in sugar lost diversity in their gut microbial communities and developed leakier guts—tight junctions in their gut walls opened up more due to inflammation from the high sugar intake.

7. Get things going; Food and beverages have been fermented by humans for thousands of years. Immunoglobulins, antibacterial peptides, antimicrobial proteins, oligosaccharides,

lipids and short amino acid sequences are all activated during the fermentation process (depending on the food). Antioxidant, hypotensive, antimicrobial, and other bioactive effects appear to be shared by these.

8. Have fun with your pet; After playing with our furry friends, most of us have been told to wash our hands. However, it appears that keeping a pet and sharing their germs could be beneficial to our microbiomes, lowering the likelihood of developing allergies and obesity.

9. Get filthy; Growing up on a farm, for example, in a microbe-rich environment can help prevent children from developing chronic diseases later in life, according to research.

10. Eliminate artificial sweeteners; Artificial sweeteners are not good for you. They are not harmful in some studies, but a recent paper found that they alter the gut microbiome and cause glucose intolerance in some groups of people.

11. Stop doing so much cleaning (yes, really); It's big business to hate bacteria. We can douse ourselves and our homes with an endless supply of antibacterial cleaning products. It's not a good idea to eat your dinner on a dirty kitchen floor, but disinfecting your hands and work surface every five minutes isn't a bad idea either.

12. Make your life easier; It's amazing how an emotion can affect our bodies' living things. Our microbiome is impacted when we are stressed because our bodies release a cocktail of hormones to prepare us to fight, fly, or freeze. While stress helps us avoid lions in the short term, it is detrimental to our gut flora in the long run.

13. Fast Although a study in mice found that changes in the microbiome as a result of fasting were associated with increases in gut mucus (which is a good thing), numbers of goblet cells (the cells that produce mucus), and length of villi (the finger-like structures on the lining of your gut that help to absorb nutrients), it seems odd that we can help our gut flora by not eating and thus starving them. Human fasting probably has the same effect.

14. Address any infections or imbalances you may be experiencing; Our guts can be infected by a wide variety of worms, parasites, and single-celled pathogens. They may cause no symptoms at all at other times, or they may cause a great deal of trouble. For instance, it has been discovered that the protozoan Giardia has a significant impact on the flora in our gut. Here, you can learn more about parasitic infection. Overgrowth of bacteria in your small intestine—where they should be very low—can have an impact on the balance of bacteria in your large intestine, which is known as SIBO.

Recommendations for prebiotics and probiotics
Including the right prebiotics and probiotics can be very helpful
in controlling Candida overgrowth. Based on the most recent
research, the following are some suggestions:

Probiotics
Both Lactobacillus acidophilus and Lactobacillus rhamnosus:
Strains are well-known for preventing the growth of Candida
and restoring healthy gut flora. Probiotic yeast Saccharomyces
boulardii: This yeast can support gut health and reduce Candida
colonization.
Bifidobacterium bifidum: This strain is important for
preventing Candida overgrowth because it helps keep the gut
microbiome in balance.
 Probiotics with multiple strains: Products like Balance ONE
Probiotic, which use controlled-release technology to ensure
that the bacteria reach the gut and contain multiple strains, are
highly recommended.

Prebiotics
Fructo-oligosaccharides (FOS): These prebiotics can help the
gut's beneficial bacteria grow, but their use in anti-Candida
regimens is up for debate. A type of soluble fiber known as

inulin is a prebiotic that encourages the development of beneficial gut bacteria.

How to Select Probiotics

CFU Count: Probiotics should contain at least 10 to 15 billion colony-forming units (CFUs) per serving.

Diverse Strains: Select products made from a variety of strains to reap the full benefits.

Method of Administration: If you want your probiotics to survive stomach acid and reach the intestines3, you should choose them with advanced delivery systems like BIO-tract. Taking these prebiotics and probiotics into your diet can help you effectively control Candida overgrowth.

Chapter 8: Management for the Long Run and Prevention

Infections with yeast are fairly common. This is especially true for yeast infections in the vagina. However, yeast infections affect more than just the genital area. They can occur anywhere on the body, including the penis and the mouth and throat. A yeast infection is typically brought on by an excess of Candida. Candida is a group of yeasts that live on the skin naturally. In normal amounts, it is usually harmless. Fungi make up the kingdom of yeast. Keep in mind that you may simply be susceptible to frequent yeast infections or have a genetic predisposition to them. However, taking preventative measures can go a long way toward avoiding yeast infections.

1. Eating a diet low in sugar

Refined sugars and high-lactose dairy products may encourage the growth of yeast, as yeasts feed on sugars and starches. Although more research is required, eating fewer of these foods may help prevent yeast infections. In the interim, getting rid of the following things may help prevent yeast infections: foods with simple sugars in them white sand brown rice beverages, and foods that have undergone yeast fermentation Cutting out sugar and refined carbs can make you feel hungry more. As a result, one should consume more of the following: vegetables and fruits with low starch legumes, nuts, and other foods high in protein healthy oils, and fats.

2. Keeping a healthy body weight Skin folds that are larger in someone who is overweight or obese may hold heat and moisture. Yeasts thrive in this environment. Additionally, being overweight or obese raises a person's risk of developing diabetes, a condition that increases a person's vulnerability to Reliable Sources of yeast diseases.

3. **Diabetic management:** High blood glucose levels in both type 1 and type 2 diabetes encourage yeast growth. Diabetes increases the likelihood of yeast infections as a result. Diabetes patients must control their blood glucose levels to reduce this risk, which typically entails: regularly keeping an eye on their levels taking diabetes medications or insulin changing their diet.

4. **Wearing clothing that lets air in Warm, moist environments is ideal for fungi**; Choose loose clothing that is made of breathable materials to avoid yeast infections of the skin and genitals, such as cotton linen silk Fabrics that wick moisture away from the skin are a good option for exercise.

Also, after a workout, don't forget to change out of wet clothes right away.

5. Being clean and tidy Improved hygiene can aid in the prevention of yeast infections; Avoid using scented products to clean the genitals because they can irritate these delicate areas. Look for products that don't have any artificial scents or harsh chemicals in them. To get rid of any excess moisture, gently but thoroughly dry the genital area after a bath or shower. Hygiene of the urn Smegma is a natural fluid that can help lubricate the foreskin and penis head, but a buildup of smegma encourages yeast growth. This buildup can be avoided by thoroughly and frequently cleaning the penis. Hygiene at the sex The following methods lower the likelihood of yeast infections in the vagina: Do not touch because important bacteria that control fungi populations are found in the vagina. Douching can result in an imbalance in these bacteria, which can lead to an infection caused by yeast and excessive growth of fungi. Wipe from front to back to stop yeast or bacteria from spreading between the anus and vagina. Change pads or tampons frequently to help prevent infections in the vaginal area.

6. preserving good sexual health; Unless individuals use barrier protection, such as condoms, yeast infections can spread to partners through sexual activity. Sometimes, a person's penis is Reliable Source itchy after unprotected sexual contact with a person with a vaginal yeast infection. Treatment is necessary for both partners if they exhibit symptoms of a yeast infection.

7. Consuming Probiotics; The populations of fungi that cause yeast infections are controlled by beneficial bacteria. A yeast infection and an overgrowth of fungi can result from an imbalance in the numbers of beneficial and harmful bacteria. The following are some of the things that can cause a bacterial imbalance: persistent stress changes or imbalances in the hormones Utilization of Antibiotics Consuming probiotics may aid in the replenishment of the body's beneficial bacteria, thereby preventing yeast infections. Probiotic-rich foods include the following: yogurt with live cultures of bacteria foods that ferment, such as kefir kimchi kombucha a few relish a little kraut.

Maintaining A Lifestyle That Is Candida-resistant

A combination of dietary choices, lifestyle habits, and regular health practices is necessary to maintain a lifestyle that resists Candida's overgrowth. Some key strategies are as follows:

1. Diet

Avoid refined carbs and sugar because Candida thrives on sugar. You can help starve the yeast by avoiding sugary foods, refined carbohydrates, and alcohol. Increase your fiber intake because fiber aids in the maintenance of a healthy gut microbiome. Eat a lot of fruits, vegetables, nuts, seeds, and whole grains. Incorporate Foods With Antifungal Properties: Apple cider vinegar, garlic, and coconut oil all naturally have antifungal properties. Fermented foods and probiotics: Yogurt, kefir, sauerkraut, and kimchi can support a healthy balance of bacteria in the gut.

2. Gut Wellness Probiotic Supplements: To support gut health, take a high-quality probiotic supplement. Prebiotics: Good bacteria in the gut are fed by foods like asparagus, onions, garlic, and leeks. Hydration: Consume a lot of water to support overall health and assist in the elimination of toxins.

3. Habits of daily life Stress management: Your immune system can be weakened by constant stress. Engage in stress-relieving activities like yoga, deep breathing, or meditation. Regular exercise helps you maintain a healthy weight and strengthens your immune system. For optimal immune system support, aim for 7-9 hours of quality sleep each night.

4. Personal Hygiene and Care; Good hygiene practices include keeping the skin folds clean and dry to stop the growth of Candida. Quickly change out of wet clothes. Use natural, gentle personal care products instead of harsh chemicals to keep your skin's natural balance intact.

5. Regular medical examinations; Keep an eye out for any symptoms of Candida overgrowth and, if necessary, seek medical attention. Visits to the Doctor regularly: Getting regular checkups can assist in the early detection and treatment of health problems.

6. Mindful Diet Completely chew: The mouth is where proper digestion begins. Food can be better digested and absorbed by chewing it thoroughly. Mindful eating: To avoid overeating, pay attention to your body's signals of hunger and fullness.

7. Avoid overusing antibiotics. Take Antibiotics Carefully: Your gut microbiome can be disrupted if you take antibiotics more often than prescribed by your doctor. You can lessen the likelihood of Candida overgrowth and improve your overall health by incorporating these strategies into your daily routine.

Chapter 9: Recent Studies On Candida

The most recent advancements in Candida research are as follows:

1. Genetic insights into the evolution of Candida Hundreds of genes in six Candida species that have recently undergone selection have been identified by researchers from the Barcelona Supercomputing Center and the Institute for Research in Biomedicine (IRB Barcelona). This study highlights both known and novel genetic variants associated with drug resistance1 and sheds light on the molecular mechanisms by which Candida pathogens adapt to humans.

2. Candida auris: A New Danger The multidrug-resistant yeast Candida auris continues to present significant clinical difficulties. The urgent requirement for new therapeutic and preventative agents has been emphasized by recent studies. Multiple distinct clades of C. auris have been identified, each with distinct clinical and microbiological characteristics.

3. Natural Treatments for Candida; A natural compound found in many plants can inhibit the growth of drug-resistant Candida fungi, including Candida auris, according to a study that was published in ACS Infectious Diseases. There may be new treatments for Candida infections as a result of this discovery.

4. Candida-Response Immunity; Type-3 innate lymphoid cells (ILC3), a subset of rare lymphoid cells, are implicated in the development of a potent immune response against Candida, according to Weizmann Institute of Science research.

New approaches to strengthening the immune system's defenses against fungal infections could be based on this finding. These updates reflect ongoing endeavors to better comprehend and combat Candida infections. Since the common fungal infection can cause a great deal of discomfort for patients all over the world, new treatments for candidiasis are extremely important. Candidiasis, which is caused by the yeast candida, can even have serious effects on people whose immune systems are weak. Global Data reports that 145 clinical trials investigating the disease have been conducted since January 2022, with another 46 planned and 19 ongoing. As new drug-resistant strains of the disease emerge, these trials gain in significance. The prevalence of candidiasis varies depending on various demographic and geographic factors. There are numerous variants. Overall, variants of Candida albicans are the most common, but regional variations of C glabrata, C tropicalis, and C parapsilosis can be more common. The disease can be treated with topical over-the-counter treatments or prescription azoles, including suppositories, when it is non-invasive and only affects mucosal surfaces or superficial skin layers. On the other hand, invasive candidiasis can result in serious, even fatal consequences. The fungus can spread to attack the eyes, heart, and kidneys, necessitating cautious primary treatment with echinocandins supplemented with fluconazole or amphotericin B administered intravenously. However, due to drug-resistant strains of the disease, the limited tissue penetration of some antifungals, and the potential toxicity of drug interactions, such treatment can become complicated. A deeper comprehension of candidiasis is necessary, as is the testing of additional novel treatments, for patients to experience the best possible recovery. What influences the spread of candidiasis? In areas of South and Central America where there are insufficient infection controls and limited healthcare resources, invasive candidiasis is common. The rate of infection varies in other parts of the world. Thailand has a higher incidence rate than Malaysia in Asia. There are more cases in Hungary than in Germany, Belgium, or Portugal in Europe. The risk of developing invasive candidiasis appears to differ by demographic. Black and African American people in the United States, along with the elderly and immunocompromised, are disproportionately affected by the fungal infection. More research is required to comprehend these discrepancies, particularly in light of the rising prevalence of non-albicans candida spp., azole resistance, and the emergence of candida auris.

Funding For Novel Treatments For Candidiasis

More than 200 clinical trials investigating candidiasis have been initiated by the global biotech and biopharmaceutical industry over the past six years, according to a recent report by Novotech, a leading contract research organization (CRO). Over sixty percent of trials are conducted in the Asia-Pacific region, primarily in China. The majority of these are Phase I trials, indicating an emphasis on preliminary research. With a wider range of Phases I, II, and III trials, countries with well-developed pharmaceutical markets like the United States, Germany, and Belgium are making significant contributions elsewhere. However, the Asia-Pacific region outpaces Europe and North America with a compound annual growth rate (CAGR) of over 20%. These figures show how much more important that area is to the development of medical research and patient care. Public institutions like the US National Institutes of Health (NIH) and the Biomedical Advanced Research and Development Authority (BARDA) are in charge of funding research into candidiasis and the development of antifungals. The United States and China are the most frequently invested in countries in the venture capital industry. The rising number of Series B and C rounds, with an emphasis on the preclinical stages to develop novel, ground-breaking treatments, demonstrates the common commitment to combating candidiasis. The most recent developments in antifungal drugs bode well for the treatment of candidiasis in the future. Brexafemme, which was approved in 2021, and Vivjoa, which was launched in 2022 to treat recurrent vulvovaginal candidiasis, both focused on vaginal candidiasis. Rezzayo also introduced a ground-breaking new treatment for invasive candidiasis in 2023. The search for a licensed antifungal vaccine continues, even as these individualized treatments cater to distinct patient requirements. Various strategies are being used in clinical trials to continue this work, including small molecules like Cresemba, which are currently leading Phase III trials. The world will benefit from improved protection against candidiasis and innovative new treatment options as vaccine development continues.

Conclusion

In conclusion, the goal of **"Candidiasis Solution: A Comprehensive Guide to Understanding and Managing Yeast Overgrowth"** was to produce a resource that was both comprehensive and useful for anyone who has been affected by Candida infections. You can take charge of your health and work toward a life free of Candida by comprehending the condition, taking a holistic approach to treatment, and staying up to date on the most recent research. We appreciate you joining us on this journey, and we wish you the best in your efforts to improve your health and well-being. We have looked at the many different aspects of Candida infections. This book aims to be a comprehensive and evidence-based resource for managing Candida overgrowth, from recognizing the various symptoms to navigating the complexities of diagnosis and treatment. The significance of gut health, the role of diet, and the advantages of incorporating prebiotics and probiotics into daily routines have all been discussed. We have also talked about changes to your lifestyle and the most recent research updates to help you take control of your health.

Understanding Candidiasis

Is Critical Anyone who has candidiasis must have a solid understanding of the condition. Overgrowth of Candida can have a significant impact on one's quality of life, resulting in a variety of symptoms that can be physically and emotionally taxing. You will be better able to recognize the symptoms of candidiasis, seek appropriate medical care, and implement efficient treatment plans if you acquire a comprehensive understanding of the condition. In the case of Candida, knowledge is power, and it is the key to regaining control of your health.

Management from all perspectives

A comprehensive approach is required for the successful management of Candida's overgrowth. This book has stressed the significance of incorporating dietary and lifestyle modifications into medical treatments. The reduction of Candida populations is greatly aided by medical interventions like antifungal medications. However, these treatments may only provide temporary relief if they do not address underlying factors like diet and lifestyle. You can create an environment that is less favorable to Candida's overgrowth and more supportive of overall health by adopting a comprehensive strategy that includes dietary modifications, stress management, and regular exercise. Knowledge as a tool for empowerment

This book's primary objective has been to equip you with the knowledge you need to make educated health decisions. You can take proactive measures in managing your condition if you are aware of the intricate nature of Candida infections, from their causes to their treatments. This empowerment involves making lifestyle choices that support long-term health and well-being rather than just managing symptoms. You will be able to confidently navigate the challenges of candidiasis and work toward achieving a life that is both balanced and healthy if you are well informed.

Research and Future Plans

There are always discoveries and advancements being made in the field of Candida research. The genetic mechanisms of Candida, the emergence of drug-resistant strains like Candida auris, and the potential of natural compounds to combat these infections have all been the subject of recent research, as we have discussed. For both patients and healthcare professionals, it is essential to remain informed about these developments. Improved treatments and preventative measures for Candida overgrowth are a likely outcome of future research, which holds the promise of improving our ability to manage it. Assistance and Inspiration It is essential to keep in mind that you are not the only one dealing with Candida overgrowth if you are experiencing symptoms right now. There are a lot of people who face similar difficulties, and there are a lot of resources and support available. Although managing candidiasis can be a journey, it can also lead to improved health and well-being if the right information and strategies are used. The goal of this book is to give you the information and tools you need to succeed on this journey. Keep in mind that you can achieve your health objectives with persistence dedication and effective management. As we come to the end of this comprehensive guide, I encourage you to put the strategies and information we've covered into practice. Changing your diet, including probiotics and prebiotics, practicing stress management, and leading a healthy lifestyle are all steps that can have a big impact on your health. Additionally, individualized guidance is invaluable in managing Candida's overgrowth, so seek professional medical advice whenever necessary. You can live a healthier life while being resistant to Candida by taking preventative measures and staying informed.

IF YOU GOT VALUE FROM THIS BOOK, KINDLY DROP A POSITIVE REVIEW FOR ME ONLINE.
https://www.amazon.com/author/elvygraves